HOW TO MANAGE YOUR EMOTIONS

Tips on how to overcome and manage negative emotions

TABLE OF CONTENT

Table of Contents

INTRODUCTION 6

CHAPTER ONE 10

8 Examples of Negative Emotions 10

Outrage 11

Disturbance 12

Dread 13

Uneasiness 14

Bitterness 15

Blame 16

Disregard 16

Depression 17

CHAPTER TWO 20

Three stages that can help you handle negative feelings 20

Stage 1: Identify the Emotion 20

Stage 2: Take Action 24

Stage 3:Get Help with Difficult Emotions 29

CHAPTER THREE 32

4 basic steps to develop positive feelings.................................32

CHAPTER FOUR 36

Step by step instructions to OVERCOME NEGATIVE FEELINGS...........36

1. Quit Justifying...36

2. Quit Making Excuses 37

3. Begin Taking Responsibility...38

4. Surpass Other People's Opinions 39

5. Stop Your Negative Habits and Avoid Bad Influences.................40

6. Think Before You Respond 41

7. Be Grateful 43

8. Eliminate impossibility From Your Vocabulary 43

9. Just Let Go 44

CHAPTER FIVE...46

Basic hints to manage negative feelings (2).............................46

CHAPTER SIX...50

5 Proven Benefits of Negative Emotions 50

1. Pity can help you focus closer on detail................................50

2. Outrage can be a solid help to look for intercession 51

3. Tension empowers better approaches for moving toward issues and difficulties...52

4. Blame causes you change negative conduct 53

5. Desire rouses you to work more diligently 54

<u>*INTRODUCTION*</u>

Feelings (emotions) are a typical and significant piece of our lives. A few feelings are good. Consider joy, euphoria, interest, inquisitiveness, fervor, appreciation, love, and happiness. These good feelings feel better. Negative feelings — like jealousy, fear, disappointment, sadness, pity, outrage, loneliness, envy, self-analysis, or dismissal — can be troublesome, even difficult on occasion.

That is particularly evident when we feel a negative feeling time after time, too firmly, or we harp on it excessively long.

Negative feelings are difficult to maintain a strategic distance from, however, everybody feels them occasionally. They might be troublesome, yet we can figure out how to deal with them.

It very well might be difficult to accept, yet feelings can become propensities that have been shaped through reiteration. Accordingly, negative feelings can become something that invades your regular daily existence.

Do you find that you're continually down on things that surround you and yourself? Do you get irritated effectively and turn out to be unpleasant with individuals? Is outrage your common reaction to something? On the off chance that you addressed 'yes' to any of these inquiries, you might be a captive to negative feelings. You need to figure out how to stop before you really change into something horrible.

CHAPTER ONE

8 Examples of Negative Emotions

Negative feelings are totally ordinary. Without them, we wouldn't have the option to value positive ones. Simultaneously, in the event that you discover you reliably have an inclination towards one specific feeling – particularly a negative one – it merits investigating why that may be.

The following are 8 normal negative feelings and why they may emerge:

<u>Outrage</u>

At any point have somebody reveal to you not to accomplish something you need? How does that cause you to feel? Does your blood start to heat up, your temperature rise and do you allegorically 'see red'? This is usually how outrage is depicted. Your body is responding to things not turning out well for you, and it's an endeavor to attempt to amend that.

Frequently when we're irate we'll yell, our face will enlist our resentment and we may even toss things around. We're attempting to get our own particular manner in a circumstance and this is the lone way we can think how. In case you're regularly responding to situations thusly, it's a smart thought to investigate why and devise more certain techniques.

Disturbance

Do you have a partner who maybe talks too boisterously? Does your partner consistently leave their messy dishes in the sink? Despite the fact that we may like our associate and love our partner, these practices can cause us to feel truly irritated. Inconvenience is the more fragile type of outrage.

While not as serious as outrage, it's the aftereffect of a comparative perspective – something has occurred or somebody is accomplishing something you wish they wouldn't. Furthermore, you have no power over it.

Dread

Dread is frequently referred to as one of the center essential feelings, and that is on the grounds that it's intensely connected with our self-appreciation protection. It's a developed reaction to caution us about hazardous circumstances, unforeseen obstructions or disappointments. We don't feel dread to feel bothered, despite what might be expected, it's there to assist us with exploring potential peril effectively.

Accepting the feeling of dread and investigating why it emerges can assist you with setting yourself up proactively to handle difficulties.

Uneasiness

Similar as dread, tension tries to caution us about likely dangers and perils. It's frequently seen as a negative feeling as it's suspected having a restless manner disables judgment and our capacity to act.

<u>**Bitterness**</u>

At the point when you miss a cutoff time, get a terrible evaluation, or don't get that work you had your expectations nailed to, you'll most likely feel pitiful. Trouble happens when we are disappointed with ourselves, our accomplishments or the conduct of another person around us. Pity can be acceptable to encounter as it shows to us that we enthusiastic about something. It tends to be an incredible impetus to seek after change.

Blame

Blame is an intricate feeling. We can feel this according to ourselves and past practices that we wish hadn't occurred, yet additionally comparable to what our conduct means for people around us. Blame is regularly alluded to as a - moral feeling and can be another solid impetus to urge us to make changes in our day to day existence.

Disregard

Like blame, unresponsiveness can be a perplexing feeling. On the off chance that you've lost eagerness, inspiration or interest in the things you've recently appreciated, this could be identified with detachment. Like annoyance, it can emerge when we let completely go over a situation or circumstance yet as opposed to losing control, we seek after a more aloof forceful articulation of disobedience.

Depression

At any point attempted to accomplish a specific assignment or objective on different occasions and not succeeded? Did that cause you to want to toss your hands noticeable all around, and outdoors in bed with an enormous tub of frozen yogurt for organization? That is gloom and it's a feeling that emerges when we aren't getting the outcomes we need. Gloom gives us a pardon to abandon our ideal objectives and it returns to a self-protection strategy.

Despondency can really be a helpful suggestion to take a break and reestablish, prior to proceeding to seek after a difficult objective.

CHAPTER TWO

Three stages that can help you handle negative feelings

Stage 1: Identify the Emotion

Figuring out how to see and recognize your sentiments takes practice. Notwithstanding zeroing in on your emotions, check in with your body, as well. You may feel body sensations with specific feelings — maybe your face gets hot, for instance, or your muscles tense.

- <u>Be mindful of how you feel</u>. At the point when you have a negative feeling, like displeasure, attempt to name what you're feeling.

For instance:

- That woman. Mary, in my group project makes me so distraught!

- I get so desirous when I see that young lady with my ex.

- <u>Don't shroud how you feel from yourself</u> You might not have any desire to communicate your sentiments to others (like your ex, for instance, or that woman in your group project who is making you frantic). However, don't smother your sentiments completely. Essentially naming the inclination is significantly better compared to claiming not to have it — or detonating without speculation.

• <u>Know why you feel the manner in which you do</u>. Sort out what happened that made you feel the manner in which you do.

For instance: At whatever point we do aggregate activities, Mary figures out how to assume all the praise for others' work.

At the point when I see my ex playing with others, it advises me that I actually have affections for her.

- <u>Don't fault</u>. Having the option to perceive and clarify your feelings isn't equivalent to reprimanding a person or thing for the manner in which you feel. Your ex presumably isn't seeing another person as an approach to get back at you, and the woman who assumes acknowledgment for your work probably won't understand what she is doing. The feeling may just be to you alone. Your sentiments are there for an explanation — to help you sort out what's happening.

- <u>Accept every one of your feelings as common and justifiable.</u> Try not to pass judgment on yourself for the feelings you feel. It's not unexpected to feel them. Recognizing how you feel can help you proceed onward, so don't be no picnic for yourself.

Stage 2: Take Action

Whenever you've handled what you're feeling, you can choose if you need to communicate your feeling. At times it's sufficient to simply acknowledge how you feel, yet different occasions you'll need to improve.

- <u>Think about the most ideal approach to communicate your feeling</u>. Is this when you need to tenderly face another person? Talk over the thing you're feeling with a companion? Or then again work off the inclination by going for a run?

For instance:

It will not tackle anything to show my outrage to Mary — it might even cause her to feel more predominant! In any case, my sentiments reveal to me that I need to try not to get in another circumstance where she assumes responsibility for a task.

- <u>Learn how to change your state of mind</u>. At one point, you'll need to move from a negative state of mind into a positive one. In any case your reasoning may stall out on how terrible things are, and that can drag you down into feeling more regrettable. Have a go at doing things that fulfill you, regardless of whether you don't feel like it at that point. For instance, you probably won't be in the temperament to go out after a messed up relationship, yet taking a walk or watching an entertaining film with companions can lift you out of that negative inclination.

• <u>Build positive feelings</u>. Good sentiments make a feeling of joy and prosperity. Make it a propensity to notice and zero in on what's acceptable in your life — even the easily overlooked details, similar to the recognition your father gave you for fixing his table or how extraordinary the food you made for lunch tastes. Seeing the beneficial things in any event, when you're feeling awful can help you move the enthusiastic equilibrium from negative to good.

- <u>Seek uphold</u>. Discussion about how you're feeling with a confided in grown-up, or a companion. They can assist you with investigating your feelings and give you a better approach for contemplating things. What's more, nothing encourages you feel more comprehended and really focused on than the help of somebody who loves you for what your identity is.

- <u>Exercise</u>. Active work helps the mind produce characteristic synthetic substances that advance a positive mind-set. Exercise likewise can deliver pressure development and help you from remaining stuck on negative sentiments.

<u>Stage 3: Get Help with Difficult Emotions</u>

Now and then, regardless of what you do, you can't shake an intense feeling. In the event that you end up stuck in sensations of trouble or stress for in excess half a month, or on the off chance that you feel so steamed that you figure you may hurt yourself or others, you may require additional assistance.

Converse with a confided in grown-up or specialist. Instructors and specialists are prepared to show individuals how to break out of negative feelings. They can give heaps of tips and

thoughts that will help you feel much improved.

<u>CHAPTER THREE</u>

4 basic steps to develop positive feelings

- **Listen to your #1 music or watch a couple of clasps of your number one humorists or motion pictures.** Thusly, you will promptly move your negative inclination states to positive feelings, for example, joy and bliss.

- **Have a discussion with a companion or somebody you realize who is known for their

humor, or positive disposition. Being in their presence will definitely have an inspiring impact on how you're feeling at the time.

• **Carry out an arbitrary thoughtful gesture.** At the point when we effectively help other people, we look outside ourselves to offer somebody help or backing, which thusly offers us a significant snapshot of direction and importance through providing for other people. Frequently, we basically need a psychological break from our own issues thus, by offering our liberality, we are helping other people in their period of scarcity, giving us a feeling of fulfillment and satisfaction.

·   **Take opportunity to do some profound breathing activities.** Profound breathing activities help by loosening up the brain and body, removing us from our pressure mode and furnishing us with much-required medical advantages all the while.

CHAPTER FOUR

Step by step instructions to OVERCOME NEGATIVE FEELINGS

1. Quit Justifying

Initially, you need to quit advocating blowing up and irritated with everything. Quit imagining that you're qualified for be so negative, since you're definitely not. The lone individual answerable for this is you.

On the off chance that you quit defending your pessimism to yourself you will not have motivation to be irate, and significantly more individuals will really appreciate being around you.

2. Quit Making Excuses

You need to quit rationalizing both yourself as well as other people. Maybe you support your own activities and why it's alright for you to express your outrage. Or on the other hand perhaps you make clarifications concerning why others merit your resentment. In any case, you're attempting to develop a socially worthy clarification for your conduct. The lone issue is that it likely isn't satisfactory and everything its doing is keeping your negative feelings alive and making you hopeless meanwhile. At last there will be nobody left to mind except for yourself. Quit making yourself a casualty. Truly consider whether these others have really done anything incorrectly.

3. Begin Taking Responsibility

Since you've quit rationalizing, it's an ideal opportunity to assume some liability for yourself and your activities. When you do this, you will begin denying your negative feelings of the force they hold over you. Own your issues and your activities and quit accusing others.

4. Surpass Other People's Opinions

Try not to let anybody however yourself characterize your mental self-view and self-esteem. This is significant, however in the event that you characterize yourself through others, you are undeniably bound to be hopeless. This is on the grounds that when you hear anything negative, you're probably going to respond with outrage and humiliation. You'll feel embarrassed and second rate and may even start enjoying self-centeredness that could prompt gloom. The joke will be on you however, on the grounds that much of the time, individuals who caused you to feel this way will not understand it. They're occupied with their own lives. The entirety of the antagonism and hurt really comes from you. You need to quit focusing on what others think right away. You'll be a lot more joyful for it.

<u>5. Stop Your Negative Habits and Avoid Bad Influences</u>

A few propensities and individuals absolutely and essentially cut you down. It could be hard to do, yet you need to eliminate these things from your life. Try not to stay nearby individuals who are negative constantly. All things considered, encircle yourself with cheerful and positive individuals who rejoice in light of life. You'd be amazed how effectively their perspectives can come off on you. Moreover, don't participate in conduct that may drive you crazy and discouraged. In the event that that bar will negatively affect you, you don't need to go there.

6. Think Before You Respond

Before you make that move, quiet yourself down.

You might be in a circumstance where your common response is to holler or send an aloof forceful message. Stop. Just, stop. Presently think. Is this something you truly need to do? Is it really that awful? Is it even worth being irate or agitated with? Did the individual you're going to respond to really do anything incorrectly, or is it in your mind? What are a portion of the potential outcomes of these activities? Will it obliterate a fellowship?

These are only a portion of the inquiries that you need to begin posing to yourself before you respond contrarily to something. You may simply find that you're thankful that you considered everything prior to acting.

7. Be Grateful

Rather than continually considering things not functioning admirably in your, begin being appreciative. What are the things or individuals you have in your life that you can be grateful for? Begin characterizing your life by the great, instead of the terrible. Start by considering at any rate one thing ordinary that you're appreciative for.

8. Eliminate impossibility From Your Vocabulary

This is a straightforward one. Saying "I can't" to things, including relinquishing negative feelings, will make it an inevitable outcome. You can't on the grounds that you say you can't. Quit setting limits on yourself and give yourself some credit. You can in the event that you say you can. Except if it's something like plunging out of a plane without a parachute and thinking you'll endure. You presumably can't do that.

9. Just Let Go

Above all, you need to attempt to relinquish your negative feelings. Clutching them and hence applying them to each seemingly insignificant detail that turns out badly isn't sound. Indeed, it's perilous. A lot of contrary individuals don't have the foggiest idea how to feel much else and aren't fulfilled except if they have something to whimper about. Unexpectedly, they're unsettled except if they're troubled and really go searching for strife. Would you truly like to be that individual? In the case of nothing else, it sounds debilitating. Release it, you will be happy you did.

CHAPTER FIVE

Basic hints to manage negative feelings (2)

The accompanying basic hints will assist you to manage negative feelings:

- **<u>Don't make a huge deal about things</u>** by going throughout them on numerous occasions in your brain.

- **<u>Try to be sensible</u>** - acknowledge that terrible sentiments are sporadically unavoidable and consider approaches to cause yourself to feel much improved.

- **<u>Relax</u>** – utilize wonderful exercises like perusing, strolling or conversing with a companion.

- **<u>Learn</u>** – notice how anguish, misfortune and outrage cause you to feel, and which occasions trigger those emotions so you can plan ahead of time.

- **<u>Exercise</u>** – high-impact action brings down your degree of stress synthetic substances and permits you to adapt better to negative feelings.

- **<u>Let go of the past</u>** - continually going over negative occasions denies you of the present and causes you to feel terrible.

CHAPTER SIX

5 Proven Benefits of Negative Emotions

At the point when taken care of well, negative feelings can have demonstrated advantages for our well-creatures.

Following are a portion of the vital discoveries from the investigation for how negative feelings can profit you:

1. Pity can help you focus closer on detail

Where positive feelings signal that everything is great in our nearby climate, negative feelings alert us that there are difficulties that requires our more engaged consideration. Pity sends us the ready that something isn't right and asks us to direct our concentration toward for what valid reason this might be, what may be causing it.

2. Outrage can be a solid help to look for intercession

Outrage has been demonstrated to urge you to search out dynamic practices to address situations or individuals you've discovered dangerous however doesn't really mean through showdown or actual demonstrations.

Outrage is a solid ready that urges you to consider why somebody may be acting a specific way, and how you can deal with reestablish harmony.

3. Tension empowers better approaches for moving toward issues and difficulties

At the point when we feel on edge, we'll attempt to do anything we can not to feel that way any longer. Tension is firmly connected to our 'battle or flight' reaction, which permits your body to make energy rapidly, good to go. At the point when confronted with risky circumstances, nervousness will dominate and urge us to look for arrangements rapidly to get away from threat.

4. Blame causes you change negative conduct

Blame can be a particularly valuable feeling. It's basically our ethical compass and when it goes off, it's a decent sign that we may have acted or said something terrible to somebody we care about. It resembles our inside framework for rebuffing ourselves when we've accomplished something incorrectly.

Individuals who are more inclined to feeling regretful are less inclined to carry out wrongdoing.

5. Desire rouses you to work more diligently

Desire isn't generally noxious. It urges us to perform better, particularly when an individual accomplished an incredible outcomes, we buckle down to accomplish that equivalent outcome or better.

This is the thing that makes understudies to perform better on tests and in homework, as seeing another understudy accomplish a passing mark made it more unmistakable for them to

accomplish as well.

www.ingramcontent.com/pod-product-compliance
Lightning Source LLC
Chambersburg PA
CBHW071239240726
48654CB00009B/1129